A Yogic Perspective on the 12 Steps

Yogi Amrit Desai

KRIPALU PUBLICATIONS

A Yogic Perspective on the 12 Steps

A STUDY GUIDE

The following is a statement of the twelve steps expounded by AA and related Fellowships, with insightful commentary by Yogi Amrit Desai based on the teaching of his yogic path to transformation.

For any spiritual path to be effective, it must provide a means for transformation, a method to help us awaken from illusion into the reality of life. Practicing the principles of these twelve steps as explained by Yogi Desai is a means by which we can overcome the illusion of the self-image and its inherent pain and make a transformational shift in consciousness.

Atma JoAnn Levitt, editor

Copyright © 1993 by Kripalu Yoga Fellowship.
All rights reserved.

ISBN 0-940258-27-7
Kripalu Publications, P.O. Box 793, Lenox, MA 01240
For information about other books and tapes by Yogi Amrit Desai and about Kripalu Center for Yoga and Health write:
P.O. Box 793, Lenox, MA 01240,
or call (413) 448-3400.

~ Step One ~

We Admitted We Were Powerless Over Our Addictions And That Our Lives Had Become Unmanageable.

COMMENTARY

This system is not about forcing or creating struggle; it is about opening to the higher consciousness within and acknowledging our helplessness in the face of what our ego-mind has created.

The doorway to transformation is the clear admission: "I feel out of control." We have no power to change our lives until we first recognize that we have a problem. So the recognition that the self-image created by the ego is running us is the first task in the transformational process. The next is to realize we do not have the power to deal with it. By acknowledging that we are out of control, we prepare ourselves to receive help from a source that is higher than we can access with our own effort.

In order to access our higher source, we have to relinquish our familiar way of dealing with life by trying to control others or ourselves. Because our minds are used to playing games, we habitually use the tools of unconsciousness to try to manipulate others to get what we want. The first step acknowledges that process from a conscious perspective and moves us toward witnessing our lives without identifying so closely with our self-image.

The process whereby the ego identifies with itself and its likes and dislikes, saying "if I produce things I want, I like myself; if I produce things I don't want, I hate myself," is the working of the unconscious. The ego has a gathering power, passing on information about its likes and dislikes to the mind, which then creates the self-image with a big "I" for "Identification." I, as the ego, then believe that self-image to be who I am.

Admitting we are powerless means recognizing that we have no control when the process of unconsciousness is in motion. The familiar tools we have used—our egos, minds, and emotions—don't work. That admission instantly provides an opening to higher channels.

Opening ourselves to the source within is the opposite of attempting to establish outward control in order to fulfill addictive tendencies. Whether we try to control through setting high standards for ourselves or others, through struggling to change reality, or through unrealistic dreams for the future, we create an enormous amount of tension that we are then obligated to discharge. Usually the tension winds up being discharged through acting on our addiction, which once again reinforces our pattern.

For example, we may put a lot of emphasis on getting rid of a compulsive food addiction, focusing energy on what to eat and at the same time fighting urges to binge. That struggle temporarily allows us to suppress our desire to overeat, but the moment we remove the pressure created by such strong expectations, it backfires. In fact, our habit returns with greater force than before.

This system is not about forcing or creating struggle; it is about opening to the higher consciousness within and acknowledging our helplessness in the face of what our ego-mind has created. The problem is not what we thought it was. The problem is unconsciousness. The whole process of dealing with addiction is dealing with unconsciousness.

When we practice the following steps, it's important to be conscious of our language. With language we create images that get embedded in our consciousness, leaving their imprint at the cellular level. In short order they become our reality. We need to be aware when we say "I am powerless" that we are referring to our ego-mind. Our real selves are God in disguise. In that aspect we are infinitely powerful, and that leads to the next step.

~ Step Two ~

Came To Believe That A Power Greater Than Ourselves Could Restore Us To Sanity.

COMMENTARY

What we've been doing might be called insanity: we've been seeking comfort for a made-up self-image rather than experiencing reality.

As we admit the powerlessness of our small selves, we also create an opening to be in touch with our higher self. That happens as soon as we recognize that our self-image, the projection of our little self outward, has always felt deficient and has escaped contact with our higher self by seeking fulfillment externally. What we've been doing might be called insanity: we've been seeking comfort for a made-up self-image rather than experiencing reality.

Now we want to come back to our source, no matter how painful or difficult that may seem. The moment we align ourselves to the source within us, we feel empowered. That "greater power" is actually the source strength that has been lying hidden within us.

Through experience, we discover that the things we've pursued in life have progressively narrowed our ways of being with ourselves and our loved ones, and have cut us off from the love we've been seeking. What we imagined was our protection has instead turned out to be our imprisonment. That is craziness.

To wake up to that process is a step toward sanity. It is like a prayer, a recognition of the heart. Such prayer emerges only when we're in total despair, when we've reached the end of our rope and see no possibility for ourselves. Only when we reach the level of personal crisis—the "dark night of the soul" where there appears to be no way out—does prayer emerge.

The only means to enter the world of inner transformation is to feel sincerely that we are helpless in the ways we've been managing our lives. By shifting into another state of consciousness, we draw upon our source strength, which helps restore our perspective and self-confidence.

~ Step Three ~

Made A Decision To Turn Our Will And Our Lives Over To The Care Of God As We Understood Him.

COMMENTARY

How strange that even though God is omnipotent and present in all of life, we human beings manage to declare ourselves separate.

Whenever we are not the controller and director of our lives, God is. The moment we relinquish our ways of automatically seeking comfort from life's problems, there is nobody else to take over but the divine. Our ego-minds are the only barrier.

The divine is already actively working within us, but all that we have acquired—our concepts, beliefs, and ways of interacting with life—poses an obstruction to our manifesting the divinity that exists within us as potential. In letting go of ego, we automatically call upon a higher will, praying: "Not my will, Lord, but Thine."

Always recognize that when we say we are powerless, we are clearly talking about the self-image that got us into this mess to begin with. The self-image has no power other than what we've given it through dreams, fears, and false beliefs. As we relinquish that mistaken identity, we allow our real selves to emerge.

Empowerment does not mean that there is an external source to give us power. What gives us power is within us, inborn as divine potential. Thus, we don't need to seek outside ourselves, but rather to open, through meditation and prayer, to what is already within us. That source is greater than we ever imagined ourselves to be. To experience the transcendental force that we are, we need the trust and faith to make a leap into that dimension.

We alone retain the possibility for transforming our lives, but most people would rather feel victimized than own the responsibility for change. Being in victim consciousness disempowers us and distances us from our source, so that we refuse to handle the issues that continually resurface.

When we separate from the power within us, believing it to be outside us, we create an internal division that causes even greater tension. To avoid that tension, we yield to desires in our attempt to control our experience: suddenly, we're back with our addiction.

In reality, there is no possibility of control in life; this life is all God. If we can let go of the need to control, we merge with the divine within us. What makes us sometimes feel separate from God are the thoughts of our ego-mind. How strange that even though God is omnipotent and present in all of life, we human beings manage to declare ourselves separate.

So we use the third step to dissolve the boundaries between us and the source within. We create an inner dialogue in which we remind ourselves:

> My real self is complete in every way. The moment I see through my mistaken identity, the self-image I've labored to create, I become more and more transparent, with fewer obstructions that keep me from the inborn light of God-consciousness.
>
> As I remove obstructions, the radiance and self-luminous consciousness I am begins to shine forth. I invoke the unlimited source of power dwelling within me as I nurture my body as the temple of God. I respect and love my body, and treat it with reverence at all times.
>
> I now prepare the altar of my heart to receive the presence that was neglected while my life's priorities focused on my self-image. When all my life was given to fulfilling my self-image, I was left unfulfilled. I now recognize that the real source of fulfillment is within me.
>
> As I release my self-image, I return to my true identity, which is no other than God, the ultimate, the limitless source, the highest consciousness.

~ Step Four ~
Made A Searching And Fearless Moral Inventory Of Ourselves.

COMMENTARY

The underlying problem is our inability to face ourselves as we really are. Unable to live with ourselves, we move into compulsive behaviors to dodge the constant conflict between the dictates of our self-image and the real self we are.

Letting go of our self-image means allowing ourselves to be totally naked before others. All that we've been avoiding or representing differently to others has been an ongoing source of tension, so it must be revealed. That is the process of the fourth step.

Making a conscious list of everything we've been hiding from means being completely honest with ourselves. Much fear and tension develops out of dishonesty; to relieve that tension we may resort to compulsive, addictive behaviors that again separate us from our true selves.

We need to say to ourselves: "I relinquish all the invisible burdens I've been collecting in the name of relieving pain. In the name of relieving pain, I've only increased it, but now I clearly recognize that these self-defeating activities never resolve my problems."

Making a list of our self-deceptions and shortcomings is a starting place. We then realize that beneath such behaviors is an unconsciousness that guides the whole process.

Rather than labeling our acts "good" or "bad," we begin to look more closely at their source. That is the way of awareness. We recognize through this inventory: "Whatever I have done, even though it might be called 'bad,' is simply the product of unconsciousness. I now choose to renounce it and live instead in the light of consciousness."

When we let go of our shortcomings, without suppressing or denying them or judging them "bad" and feeling an obligation to become "good," we allow source consciousness to flow through us. "Good" is not something we have to do; it's what we already are.

When "good" is pitted against "bad," our minds trap us in the field of relativity. That means things look either relatively better or relatively worse. Once we establish change, there is often fear involved: "If I'm relatively better, I can get relatively worse." Through that kind of thinking, we're chained to dualistic awareness. In that state our creative source awareness may not surface.

We need to do more than just understand what our problem is. We may understand the problem extremely well in our minds. However, that is not the solution; the solution is in the experience of going beyond the mind. When we transcend the mind and work from beyond our limited consciousness, we uproot the entire system that created our compulsive behaviors and transform the unconscious material.

To become fully conscious, we must let go of all dualistic thought patterns that are limiting in nature. Replacing one belief with another is only relatively better, however. What we need is to engage in transformation, not reformation.

Sometimes, for example, when we have become abstinent, we have a fear of falling back into addiction. Although we have given up our primary addictive substance or behavior, we may initiate some other form of unconscious living due to the root fear of the direct experience of our inner feelings.

The underlying problem is our inability to face ourselves as we really are. Unable to live with ourselves, we move into compulsive behaviors to dodge the constant conflict between the dictates of our self-image and the real self we are. The process of recovery means letting go of the image and returning to the source within.

The purpose of this inventory, then, is not to get rid of addiction but, by returning to our source, to eradicate the whole system that gives rise to addictive tendencies. Awakening the presence of witness consciousness helps us recognize the true nature of our problems, which then don't need to be fought, struggled with, or judged. By shifting our consciousness we transcend them.

~ Step Five ~

Admitted To God, To Ourselves, And To Another Human Being The Exact Nature Of Our Wrongs.

COMMENTARY

Commitment to honesty with others helps us transcend ingrained patterns of fear and avoidance, and our dishonesty with ourselves.

In all these steps there is an underlying commitment that we make to ourselves. It is that under no circumstance will we go back to using the objects or behaviors of addiction. That commitment is absolutely necessary, because once we enter the process of healing, we will begin to feel the inevitable pain of living. Avoidance of pain is what got us into addiction. If we are still unwilling to experience the pain of living, we'll be back in the same frame of mind that brought us to the place we are now. Commitment is necessary to transcend our minds.

In the same way commitment to honesty with others helps us transcend ingrained patterns of fear and avoidance, and our dishonesty with ourselves. So we want to declare our patterns and our fear. In admitting those to others we allow ourselves to go beyond the image we've projected that we are in control of our lives, or that we are great and powerful.

Honesty with others goes hand in hand with honesty with ourselves, so it's an important part of the process. If we do not let others know who we really are, then we have no access to our source. We suppress our source strength by generating an image that we would like ourselves and others to believe. Then we deplete our precious energy maintaining that image, which essentially means struggling to maintain a pack of lies.

Declaring ourselves to others is a means of returning to source, if the admission is based upon our personal integrity. If we don't have integrity, no matter what we tell others, we'll wind up violating our own principles. What makes this step work, then, is not "sharing with others" so much as buying into it ourselves, with all our hearts, and recognizing deep within that "my life does not work when I live from my habits and conditioning." That is why we admit to God and ourselves first, before we admit to another, the exact nature of our wrongs.

~ Step Six ~
Were Entirely Ready To Have God Remove All These Defects Of Character.

COMMENTARY

Another way of stating the sixth step is "Were entirely ready to move out of the unconsciousness in which we performed past actions and into the conscious state of the higher self."

There are no real defects in us. Whatever has happened, happened to us in a particular state of consciousness. The moment we shift our consciousness, we no longer need to fight to change what went on in other states; it's totally irrelevant. We enter a whole new dimension and a whole new reality.

Although in our "waking" state we appear to be functioning on a conscious level, it is only conscious compared to the sleep state. No matter what kind of dream or nightmare we had while sleeping, once we wake up we don't need anyone to convince us that it wasn't real. It drops away because we have shifted into another state of consciousness.

In the same way, there is a state of consciousness beyond the "waking" state and that is called the "awakened" state. By surrendering to the process of transformation, we are not trying to get rid of ineffective behaviors, but, instead, are shifting into another level of consciousness altogether.

Another way of stating the sixth step is "Were entirely ready to move out of the unconsciousness in which we performed past actions and into the conscious state of the higher self." Our new, more conscious state allows us to see beyond what we had defined as "right" and "wrong" in the reality of our "waking" state. From this new state of consciousness we see that "I am only the witness, not the doer of action." The doer that identified with so-called "rights" and "wrongs" was the personality, or persona —the mask, or self-image.

Once we relinquish the protective and ego-centered self-images, we can witness them. Even though we may still judge actions as "right" or "wrong," we no longer judge ourselves for the actions of our past. Rather than attempting to change "bad" to "good," witnessing allows us to rise above them both and see them as the creation of the self that identified with them.

In the past, through identification with our addiction, we created much tension within ourselves. Now we rise above any fear of "wrong" or hankering after "right." We shift out of the unconscious state into the witness state, owning fully the consciousness of our own freedom.

This is the most ancient teaching. What this asks is that from the very beginning we recognize and construct our lives based upon the knowledge that we are born divine. Willingness to have our shortcomings removed is another way of saying we affirm the fundamental truth of our divinity and we choose to live in witness consciousness.

~ Step Seven ~
Humbly Asked God To Remove Our Shortcomings.

COMMENTARY

Letting go of ego is an invocation of God's presence, an experience of relaxation, joy, and communion with our inner source.

Who is this external God that we are asking to remove our shortcomings? The truth is that the moment we are successful in dropping the dualities the mind creates, we manifest the divine. We are God—the witness, the higher self—and we are established in that Godhood. Letting go of ego is an invocation of God's presence, an experience of relaxation, joy, and communion with our inner source.

The whole process of admitting that we are powerless, making an inventory, and asking for help to overcome our problems is a function of humility. But honestly aligning with our higher self goes beyond humility. In humility there is still the possibility of self-deception. Even in prayer, which is the ego-self's petitioning, there is the possibility of self-deception. Aligning with our higher self goes beyond humility to the honesty of the witness state, where there is no room for deception because there is nothing "bad" to fight or "good" to hanker after.

Being conscious means entering into choiceless awareness: we do not identify with "right" or "wrong," nor do we run from what we consider negative or toward what we consider positive. Such action kept us confined to the level of dualistic reality. Now our experience transforms as we move into the "awakened" state of consciousness, the state of choiceless awareness.

So to reframe the seventh step, we may say: "We recognized our true nature as the higher self, allowing the reality of our actions to be revealed and releasing any negative judgments of our minds." Letting go of what we have called shortcomings then happens without our having to ask for it. Asking reinforces the idea that "I am short of something," when the fact is that the real self is free of any shortcomings.

~ Step Eight ~

Made A List Of All Persons We Had Harmed, And Became Willing To Make Amends To Them All.

COMMENTARY

What is true in our relationship with others is also true in our relationship with our self-image, or ego-self.

As long as we live with a limited definition of reality, we reinforce our concepts. Overcoming addiction may be a first step to freedom, and carefully and realistically assessing the effects of our addictive behaviors is also essential. True freedom, though, is an experience beyond concepts. Therefore, it is important in this step to be aware of the language we give to our actions and the way that language imprints upon our consciousness.

Yogis have said "Thou art that," meaning that we are born enlightened. They say that our light has simply been covered by clouds of misconceptions. But even when we do not see the sun, the sun is still there. In the same way, consciousness, the spark of God or soul or spirit, already dwells within us. The honesty of this step of acknowledging the effects of our past actions creates an opening for us to realign with the truth of our being.

When we look at our past actions, it's important to remember Jesus' statement "Judge not, lest ye be judged," because what is true in our relationship with others is also true in our relationship with our self-image, or ego-self. Any judgment puts us back in the field of relativity. When we judge, we cut ourselves off from our witness awareness and deny the divine that is present within us.

In making this list, then, and in using it as a tool for transformation, it is vital that we are not motivated by fear or self-judgment. Our actions need to be generated instead from love and acceptance. Our motivation needs to come from a different state of being—from our love for everything that is great and divine within us.

~ Step Nine ~

Made Direct Amends To Such People Wherever Possible, Except When To Do So Would Injure Them Or Others.

COMMENTARY

By making peace with the other, we're really bridging the separateness we feel within ourselves.

Sincerity is the crucial component of the ninth step. Letting go of the need to hide ourselves or to project ourselves differently from the person we are has the vital effect of helping us become truly honest with ourselves. Everything rests in our willingness to face who we are. Going through the motions of self-disclosure won't work unless it leads to the subtle process that takes place behind those admissions to our friends.

If we go directly into the process, there is no room for self-deception. We must be willing to witness and be with ourselves as we really are. Then we are clear even as we admit our weaknesses.

This step says, "Go and admit what harm you have done to others, and make peace with yourself and with the other person. Do it from your heart, from the very depth of your being." That means we do it with a sincere desire not only to let go of the action but of the pattern that gave rise to that action and created distance between ourselves and others.

When we let go of patterns that separate us, integration automatically takes place. As we remove our distance from others, we also remove our distance from ourselves. By making peace with the other, we're really bridging the separateness we feel within ourselves.

~ Step Ten ~

Continued To Take Personal Inventory And When We Were Wrong Promptly Admitted It.

COMMENTARY

Self-observation is a meditative process in which we develop the capacity to witness all of life.

Continuing to take inventory is the process of self-observation, which means observing our lives through witness consciousness without judging or condemning ourselves. That observation needs to be done, as much as possible, on a moment to moment basis. Whether we do it silently, out loud with another, or by journaling, we admit the motivations we have avoided facing and the strategies we have used to build our image in the world.

By constant focus, we develop the habit of watching ourselves and thus learning who we are. Self-observation is a meditative process in which we develop the capacity to witness all of life, without going after what is desirable or fighting what is undesirable.

Our process of self-discovery becomes more firmly rooted as time goes on. Letting go of compulsive behavior is only one step along the way; our willingness to witness our actions and experience the many facets of who we are is the real pathway to self-knowing. Continued practice brings us the awareness that our deepening self-knowledge itself precipitates ongoing changes in our behavior.

~ Step Eleven ~

Sought Through Prayer And Meditation To Improve Our Conscious Contact With God As We Understood Him, Praying Only For Knowledge Of His Will For Us And The Power To Carry That Out.

COMMENTARY

Conscious contact brings us to the level of our soul's reality, so that we are not thinking about God, but actualizing God in each moment.

This step is the means by which we access the witness consciousness we have been talking about. In our unconsciousness we have identified ourselves as separate from the whole of creation, and that is a fallacy. We have exerted a lot of effort attempting to control our environment and to maintain that false identification with our separateness.

To heal ourselves we must move into the consciousness that "I and my God are one and the same." That is the purpose of improving conscious contact with the source within us. The more we contemplate spiritual teachings, meditating and reflecting deeply, the more we dislodge ourselves from our false identifications with our self-images and move into alignment with our true being.

One way to disengage from old images of ourselves and improve conscious contact with our source is to place a picture of ourselves beside that of a teacher whom we venerate and by meditating blend the two images. It doesn't matter what our religion is: if we feel drawn to the teachings of the Christ, we can attune to Christ consciousness; if drawn to Buddha, we can attune to Buddha consciousness. Whoever our teachers and whatever our means of inspiration, we can allow those spiritual teachings to enter and guide our prayers and meditations. In that way we achieve transcendence, using the inspiration of our chosen path.

It is important also to remember that addiction never happened to our true selves: we are the witness. Addiction happened to the self-image in its efforts to get rid of some perceived problem that never existed the way we thought it did. It was our limited self-concept that caused the problem in the first place. If addiction could happen to our real selves, then there would be no possibility of God or source.

All that is transitory happens to our transitory selves, while our real selves remain unattached and free. As we watch the passing phenomena through meditation, we learn the nature of what is transitory and what endures.

The real self is unconditional. That means it's unconditionable: it cannot be conditioned. If our soul could be affected by external changes, it would not be divine. It is said that no matter how much water you throw on a swan, it rolls off its back. The same is true of the self. In India, when a person attains that higher self, the person is called "paramahansa," which means "supreme swan." Such a person can live in this world, but is not limited by the world.

Meditation helps us access our higher power by turning our focus and concentration inward. Watching our thoughts surface while disengaging from them creates a distance and neutrality in relation to all we observe. Without meditation we could continue to be a victim of our mind's games, either expressing or suppressing unconscious urges.

Only through witnessing can we allow all that has been unconscious to come forth on a conscious level. In that way we experience a type of contact with our divinity that is very deep and sustaining. Conscious contact brings us to the level of our soul's reality, so that we are not thinking about God, but actualizing God in each moment.

~ Step Twelve ~

Having Had A Spiritual Awakening As The Result Of These Steps, We Tried To Carry This Message To Others, And To Practice These Principles In All Our Affairs.

COMMENTARY

Those whom we call addicts are simply intense seekers of bliss who have gotten stuck in repetition, looking for the right thing in the wrong place. When we let go of the self-image we used to identify with, we find behind it the experience of unity we've been seeking.

Our source is ever drawing us toward union with itself. Because of our lack of understanding, that urge toward divine bliss becomes diverted into the search for security, pleasure, and power, which can lead to addiction. Now, the addiction and the process of following these steps have been a doorway to true spiritual awakening. Since we can't simply remain in the doorway, Step Twelve invites us to move through it into a deeper awakening, using the practice of the steps, participation in a spiritual community, and the offering of loving selfless service.

Whenever we have an experience of transcendence, all the attributes of life change before our eyes. For instance, when water is liquid it seeks out lower ground, moving constantly downward. When it is transformed, it becomes vapor and moves upward. It has a totally different character. We cannot replace water with steam or steam with water; they each have a different function to fulfill.

When we speak of transcending the "waking" state, we are not denying its value or worth. The "waking" state of consciousness is necessary in order to survive on this plane. At the same time, it is important to go beyond it, because once we learn to shift our consciousness from the "waking" to the "awakened" state, we can live in this world with greater creativity and energy at our disposal.

Moreover, our experience of the "awakened" state is very different from that of the "waking" state, in which "might is right" and survival of the fittest seems the main guideline. In the "awakened state," the guideline is "blessed are the meek." On the material plane, the more we get, the more we have. On the spiritual plane, the more we give away, the more we receive.

Giving, in the "awakened" state, becomes receiving, which comes about as an overflow of the abundance of spirit. As we share our experience, strength, and hope with others, we help them experience their source and in the process reinforce our own spiritual awakening. That eventually brings us to a state of bliss, which is our natural state.

All of nature is in bliss. Trees are in bliss. Mountains are in bliss. That is what holds life together. If something is not in bliss, it is out of harmony with the universe. But although animals and all living things are in bliss, humans are the only ones who can consciously experience that bliss.

Those whom we call addicts are simply intense seekers of bliss who have gotten stuck in repetition, looking for the right thing in the wrong place. When we let go of the self-image we used to identify with, we find behind it the experience of unity we've been seeking.

With that new awareness, we no longer need to struggle with "recovery." We say to ourselves, "I am now living in a new dimension where I trust the source of power that is my sustaining grace. I am free of fear, no matter what may happen to my self-image. I live now in a state where I am showered by grace at every moment." Then we participate in life, not as a child of God, but as God himself. That is what being divine means.

Basically we have to relinquish the concept that God is outside ourselves and recognize that we are God. We are born with that divine potential, and the challenge is to discover that it is within us, not outside us. Only the source can give us freedom.

The ultimate goal of spirituality is to be free from everything and everyone, and that is the opposite of addiction. When we become free in that way, we are also free from God, because God is a concept as well. That is why yogis say "Thou art that" or "Aham Brahmasmi," which means "I am the Brahman (the Ultimate Reality)." There is no God independent of us.

The twelfth step is also about keeping supportive company and offering selfless service. Company is much stronger than will power. In Steps One through Three, we acknowledged that our minds alone were powerless to transform our lives and we surrendered to the transforming energy of higher consciousness. That higher consciousness often manifests through our experience in spiritual community. Therefore, surrounding ourselves with others on a spiritual path is fundamental to our transformation. When we participate in spiritual community, we have an opportunity to reinforce our spiritual understanding by offering loving, selfless service.

Loving service demands that we let go of manipulating others or being dishonest with others or ourselves. Loving service, then, becomes a training in non-attachment. Relinquishing our desires for external rewards or recognition in turn awakens and strengthens the inner source of our security and fulfillment.

By committing to loving service of others, we serve the divine self within, as we create the conditions in which we experience love directly, even as it is drawn from us in service to others. In the process of loving, we are the ones who are transformed.